Quit Smoking: Tell Cigarettes to Fuck Off – The Easy Way to Quit Smoking in 96 hours or less

It has been two years (1,051,200 minutes & counting) since I told smoking to FUCK OFF! I dedicate this book to my rocks and foundation Julianna, Rebecca and Melissa. Thank you for putting up with the first 5,760 minutes and so many more.

Contents

Forward

Before you start reading onwards, I am going to warn you that this is not your traditional bullshit self-help book about quitting smoking. This book is written for those brave Mother Fuckers who wants to take that next step in their life and become free from nicotine. Now it doesn't matter whether that be cigarettes, cigars or even vaping. Normally one would include gum in the group because it also contains that sweet nectar of addiction but I say go for the gum because it does not involve combustion which release all the toxins and negatives of smoking but enough of that we are getting side tracked.

I chose to write this book as short as possible for two reasons because one I am not a professional writer and two, quitting smoking isn't rocket science. As we both know there are some dumb fuckers out there that have done the impossible. Stop and take a moment to now think to yourself are they really dumber? We both know this is a rhetorical question and the answer to this question does not need to be said aloud because they aren't the poor suckers shelling out 20 percent of their paycheck each and every month since you don't have the will power to own up to your issues. That one stung and here is one of the few apologies I will give. I am truly sorry for telling you the truth but it's still the truth.

In my opinion this book will be the best $9.99 you will ever spend. Just think even buying this book is cheaper than a pack of smokes. Here are some quick questions for you. Are you tired as hell with getting winded after 50 ft jog or sick of the famous mating call of the smoker, the smokers cough? Well then this is the book for you and it is going to knock your fucking socks off. In the end, you and only you will come out with two results. In laments terms either you will quit or you don't. In the end, you are the only person responsible for those results regardless of all the fucking excuses in the world. I like to use this statement a lot, there are always excuses but is there really ever a reason.

After a long chat with my 78-year-old grandmother I asked Nan how she finally quit after smoking for 30 years? Nan being Nan said by taking each day one minute at a time and sucking it up in the will power kind of way by not putting the filter to her lips in any kind of way. At first, I was confused as there was no way it was that simple but I sat down and dwelled on this conundrum for the whole afternoon. All of a sudden, the light came on, it was dim yes but never the less it came on. It was all about minutes so I started breaking down cigarettes to numbers and then converting minutes. As some would say, real mathematical shit but in the end this boring ass math is really a method that helped me quit and leave finally leave the longest, most abusive & negative relationship of my life.

Now we are going to compare smoking to a common occurrence that we all experience. When you think about smoking, I need you picture that friend or partner who's really not a friend or a partner but is always there for you, come on, now really come on, you know the one. I need you to take all your will power and tell them after 5, 10, 20, 30, even if somehow the big C didn't get you first 50 years to go fuck off. Go fuck themselves and piss off. Tell them to take their shit and get of my life, scream take your greedy hand out of my pocket and slip that slippery knife out of your back. Let them know to take their crushing anxiety, the overwhelming weight that they give you when they are not around. Let them know passionately to take that depression. All those negative feelings they bring on when you try to leave them yet somehow someway you keep going back to them like a beaten lover. You may think that you love them, you believe that you need them and that you can't live without them. Today is the day you are going to let them know how every day they are killing you. Slowly eating away at you, adding wrinkles, receding your gums and hairlines. Go ahead and use conviction to notify them you are done with their shit. Say to them you are leaving them and in 96 hours you are done. Tell them you will pack up your lungs and being moving onwards. I know and you know that it will take years to reverse the damage you received from this association but in the end you have changed. You have made the conscious choice to live a healthier, wealthier and more successful life.

At the end of the day I guess I just want to say that this book, well this life changing, 'mind altering' book is dedicated to all the people who tried to quit people but never had the chance unlike you to quit because one of the big diseases got them either it was cancer, emphysema or heart conditions. As a former smoker who was in that abusive relationship; no really look up the definition. I was in that relationship for 22 years. I started smoking when I was in grade 5, making me just 11 years old. That year I was suspended for the first time for smoking but then again it was still cool to smoke back then. Over those 22 years I probably inhaled enough tar to pave a Costco parking lot. Look at the chemicals listed on the pack, that is just 20 of over 3000 different types. Start thinking how much of each of those toxins have you so graciously pumped into your lungs all in the name of love. The love of nicotine and paying the poor tax.

Chapter 1 – Telling Your Cigarettes to FUCK OFF

Before we officially get started here on our journey, I would like to say I'm very proud of you, your family and friends are very proud of you, even your co-workers as they will no longer have to absorb that nasty ass smell of smoke day in and day out. All this praise for accepting the second hardest challenge of your life. The first being even getting out of bed to challenge this world for all your worth. This isn't a pat me on the back kumbaya book, this is a quick, costless and efficient method to quit smoking in 96 hours or less. Now let's get some more pats on the back for you to get you motivated.

In the end most importantly your health is very proud of you because you're going to take the biggest step of your life but enough of whether we are proud, or your family's proud of you or anyone else. The only person here that needs to be proud of YOU is YOU. Now let me repeat that going through this book and through this process the only person that YOU need to make proud is YOU. The only person you can truly be doing this for is you, you can have inspirations like your kids or making you more attractive or your partner bought you this book. No matter how you slice it this mission is on you and you only. You and only you are responsible for you own outcomes. I know I am repeating myself over and over again but this phrase is very important to the process. I always emphasize with anyone I work with about quitting smoking. If you're not ready quit then you won't, let me repeat that again If **you're** not ready quit then **you** won't. I mean if you want to go out and waste your money, I will be glad to receive it because just like you I got bills to pay too but the money your throwing away should ultimately be staying in your pocket for you to pay your bills.

You are going to notice I repeat myself throughout this book many times but as a parent I have learned that if I want to help teach my kids then repetition builds understanding, it's not my quote but I know it's somebody's. I plant the idea in their head then repeat, repeat, repeat then let them come to their own conclusions. I always support them regardless but I also always let them know YOUR outcomes are the results of YOUR decisions. YOUR habits become part of your character. Certainly, as you know that smokers can act like real children when we need our little friend Puffy. Puffy makes you feel so good. We will hide in spots we are not allowed just to put Puffy to your lips. Most smokers accept no responsibility for their smoke and when you tell them about the issue just wait for the defense mechanisms. The hair on their spines stand up then the denial kicks in. They start standing up for that friend, oh nothing is coming between me and my friend. I referred to my smoking as Puffy. My relationship with Puffy was very shitty but I haven't seen the asshole in two years. They defend that Puffy has just as much right to be here as anyone else. You are getting the picture once again this masterpiece is not your regular quit smoking book. My inner Samuel is coming out of me. There're mother fuckin smokes in this mother fucking pack.

If you are taking this next step in life because somebody else wants you to quit or somebody else bought you this book thinking subliminally you might just pick it up? If you answered yes to either of these questions then put this book down now and just walk away. Don't put yourself including your mind, body and nerves through the agony and suffering, don't make the people you love go through the hostility either even though they should have suffer to as well, those horrible evil people who love me so much they want me to live longer So we can enjoy our lives together or even to put more food on the table (we all have a smoke budget). How much is yours $100, $200, $300, let me ask you a question out loud. Have you ever chosen cigarettes over food? If you have, can please sit down and really think for a moment what the fuck has been wrong with me? Don't feel bad we all have done the same; it sucks but that is the nature of addiction.

If YOU are not ready to quit then you are not going to quit no matter how little or how much effort you put in. This is a one-person game and quote 2Pac "It's just me against the world". Through this journey you are going to be amazed at the number of jerks that suddenly show up in your day whether it be at the store or in traffic. You will notice people who just agitate you all along the way. Either their knee is rocking, they're chewing too loud or I can hear the clicking of their teeth. All we can say is you just wait until day 3 when you want to kill every single smiling person there is on the way to work but Don't worry trust me these are basic human reactions we feel when you decide to completely detox your body of nicotine. Every person who has ever quite smoking, at least thought of murdering a few people through their voyage over broken glass. These things are always going to happen. I must warn you that if you are not committed then please put down this book for now and come back to it when you are ready, in saying so however there is still a ton good shit in this book to read so feel free to continue.

Over my many minutes on this earth I have learned if there's any one thing you can do for your body it would be to get rid of those cancer sticks. They will both physically and psychologically make you it's bitch. At the end of the day; you know what fuck it and eat the red meat, eat that big juicy hamburger, it's still healthier than putting over 3000 chemicals into your lungs every day. Growth hormones over formaldehyde any day. Jaywalk when there is no traffic. Don't wear condoms, I bet that by adding up all the STIs together, less people still die than from government sponsored smoking programs every year, and lastly forget to stretch when you work out tonight. Almost anything you do if safer for you than smoking, I repeat almost anything. I am not endorsing any of these activities just listed, I am just trying to point out how totally fucking stupid smoking really is, I makes no sense to spend all my money to kill myself. Sure it was cool when we were young but the year is 2019 and the times have changed. Joe Camel probably died and how come we never hear what happened to the Marlboro Man. Uh, Uh… Cancer.

Here is my oath to you. I, Joel Young, swear to God, Buddha, whatever tickles your fancy or even the little atoms floating around in front of me, that I openly and honestly swear to YOU (insert your Name) that choosing to quit smoking is the single best decision of your life. Because cancer usually lasts a lifetime. I look back my decisions and I see all the wonderful things I have had the chance to experience and all the things I know I am now going to have unless I get hit by a bus, you know what though, I still like the bus odds better than smoking.

Now stop and take 1 a few minutes to yourself and think deeply about what have been the best decisions of your life. Now that you have thought about it, which choices of freewill brought you happiness? Now I getting ready to hear the answers and be honest here, don't give me that regular fluff that the happiest day of my life was when I got married (Your spouse isn't here) or my kid was born (you kids aren't lurking around the corner like Michael Myers on Halloween, or when I got that promotion because your boss doesn't really care. These are the all best decisions as of yesterday. These were all great but think of how much more tomorrow's decision is going to change your life when you tell smoking to fuck off. Tomorrow morning when you wake up you will have the all-time best decision of your life. Now just think of this who have you been married to longer your partner of the 15 years or that old partner who keeps following you around you know old faithful Puffy, no matter where you go there, Puffy was there, you can't live without them. But not anymore you are making the decision to live your life for yourself and not for nicotine.

I guarantee you that if you follow the steps that I gave you in this book and you truthfully go the 96 hours you will have quit smoking you. End of story. By following the steps when you have quit smoking you can please contact us at U and Me Publishing so we can hear your success story. If this book doesn't work then we will send you back the money that you paid for this book but you have to honestly say did I try and admit you are not just trying to get your money back because you are too weak to go for a new life for you.

As we both know you can only give a person the tool and let them figure it out. I can only help you reach YOUR outcome; this is on you and only you so get ready to suck it up, oops sorry I guess that would be the wrong expression, here is a new one you probably haven't heard before "get ready to quit sucking it up and start telling nicotine to Fuck Off". That's right take their dopamine induced pleasure and go fuck itself.

Chapter 2 – Scaring the Shit out of You

Let's face the facts of life, we are all going to die at some point as no one can outlive the reaper. Another interesting fact is that there is one universal currency every human possesses. Every person is born on day one with an equal bank account before considering any other outside factors like race, socio-economic, or etc. get applied. We all have the same bank account from the same institution and they further provide an account of time which as the days go by will contain debits and credits of minutes. How we use our time completely depends on each of us independently. We use our time to carry out activities or choices throughout our lifetime which in return they either increase our chances of death or inversely, decrease your chances. Either way those particular choices fall on your shoulders and you are the only variable whom controls those chances. Further for those people out there, yes there are somethings that you have absolutely no control over like involved or uninvolved third parties or so called "acts of god". For the purpose of this lecture or rant or whichever you want to call it, we don't give a single fuck about them from now on, we only give a shit about us and our success, we give zero fucks to what we can't control so we are going to push aside all of it and let fate playout. We will simply let nature take its course.

Worrying about what you can't control will destroy you from the inside out, my advice is to always move forward with zero fucks given. Give your fucks to those occasions that really deserve them and when you are quitting smoking it's the little things that are what won't let you quit smoking. All those tiny things, the drip of the water or the glass being in the wrong place, the boss speaking to you about an issue with your work, and then you end up quitting the quitting process. They eat at you and they nag at your very soul until you crave that sweet relief. "It's just one it won't hurt nothing, a quickie out back behind the bush with Puffy" but you are hiding out there because you are ashamed that people might see you being weak and not stick true to the new you. Your cheating already.

In the end its still really only your decision to put the cigarette to your lips, nobody is holding you down and forcing you to smoke it. Christ those things are fucking expensive to begin with so why in the world would somebody hold you down and force you to smoke them. Come on now give me another excuse why your arm was twisted so hard. Now to control that universal back account, one can go for it all in life leaving no risk unchecked or apply some risk management control over their own choices, like either quitting smoking or not walking into traffic but in the end our clocks only have so many minutes. So, let me ask this question. As of today, is how are you (Insert Your Name) going to use those minutes? Are we going for the red or the black, the blue pill or the red pill, heads or tails?

This is the fun chapter; this is chapter in which I will probably bore the living hell out of you, so please feel free to skip ahead if you already feel comfortable in knowing how fucked up smoking really is but in case you don't then I want to bring you face to face with some scary statistics. After reviewing countless reports and articles, from sources such as the CDC Center for Disease Control, the National Cancer Institute, the World Cancer Research Fund, the list goes on and on. Literally google the term quitting smoking you will receive over 95 million web pages in a 0.47 second search, jeepers how much for a full minute search? When it comes to smoking after looking at the facts, it leads one down the yellow brick road to the conclusion of a gigantic pile of bad shit where everyone is dying and everyone is sick or poor.

All I am really doing each day is taking or adding minutes from my life. As a client of life dipping into my bank account existence. When I am smoking, I am using up my currency by debiting the account and we both know absolutely nothing good comes out of. It doesn't matter where you are from, neither gender, nor form of spiritual belief, it really doesn't make too much of a difference to any demographic because in the end smoking usually ends the same way. Somebody is either sick or dead, I have never heard of anyone getting healthier besides the smokers who use the excuse. You know one of the most lame ass excuses, "I was so sick when I tried to quit" or "I had headaches and chest pains". Well no shit, that side effect is called withdrawal. Can you honestly tell me one good result of cigarettes? Now before you answer that question sit down and really think about all the wonderful benefits you are gaining.

Either way it's very easy to tell you that I hate cigarettes. I believe they are the devil if there is one and if not then a tool of the evil bastard himself. There are no other utensils to explain the conundrums of nicotine addiction outside of adultery which is usually free by the way. Tobacco is a solid number for the ultimate test of freewill. You will be tested so frequently you will feel like you went from kindergarten to 12 in just a day now let's get our asses moving on and butting out.

As we talked about in chapter one this book is about breaking up with Puffy. The first two stats we look at are (A) which is how long have you have been committed to this one-sided abusive relationship or in other words when you took your first puff. The moment you put those sweet virgin lips on Puffy. The second stat (B) which is the age when you first tried to quit and leave the miserable fucker. You could see the negative effects even then but oh how they have been there. Every time you tried to quit since the situation arises and all of sudden there you are back putting your lips on their dirty old butt, god knows what types of gases we are breathing in today.

Now look at those numbers, there is no need to feel depressed just realize that this is how long you have been putting up with the addiction of nicotine. So, let me ask again, how long you have been trying to escape their clutches? I bet you tried and tried again but as the years went on, they just kept digging their clutches deeper into you until now it has become a part of you and your identity. You have become engrained as a person. An identity that as of today or tomorrow is no longer you and will never be you again. Fuck Off, Puffy Fuck Off. Every day is a new day and each great thing was accomplished with just one a step and or just a minute of your time. You heard me just quit, you can do it and you know it. The only one person who can stop for you is you. If I can quit then anyone can. It's a one-person game.

Now since statistics and numbers really don't lie, math is the universal language similar to time being our universal currency, math doesn't change no matter where you are in the known proven universe. The equation 1 plus 1 equals 2 or 6 times 6 equals 36 are both the same on Earth and Uranus but back to the point, below is my super-secret formula. Here is the simple formula for figuring it out how many smokes you pumped into your one and only set of lungs over your life time:

X (# Years) * Y (Avg. # Cigarettes/day) * 365 = Estimate of the number of smokes you have had in lifetime.

Let's break this down, take the amount of years you have been smoking, which is called X then multiply X by the Y which represents the average amount cigarettes you smoke in day then multiply the end result by 365 days. The final result will be how many individual times you have sat done with Puffy. How many intimate moments have you had? How many cigarettes you have suffered through?

Now let's go to beyond and look at how much time, I mean actual time you have spent with that fucker. Now let's assume the average cigarette takes around two minutes to smoke. We further know the truth if there are no other likeminded individuals killing themselves with you then you are going to get it into to you as quick as possible. Enough of that now let's take the answer from the first equation and multiply that number by 2 which represents 2 minutes. The answer is that's how many minutes of your life you have physically spent putting Puffy's dirty tip in your mouth. Yes, because guess what you are getting fucked daily and not in the good way. Let's go even further into the ever-exciting world of math now I hate math too but when it's this easy to see. You will know why by the end of day four why two minutes is not worth it.

Let's take those numbers even further by taking the total number of minutes and divide it by 60 representing one hour. That's how many hours physically you have spent smoking, now let's dive peeper go ahead and divide that number by 24 that is how many days, and you can go so forth and so forth. Please now take a moment to yourself, and truly digest those numbers. Math won't lie unlike a smoker looking for an excuse. How much of your life was spent with Puffy, just you and them? In the rain, in the cold, in the snow and ice and I am not even a postal employee. On a sidewalk or in a basement, it doesn't matter it's just the two of you and the time you spend together.

At this point, just so you truly see how stupid smoking is, go ahead and see how many actual days of your life. How many full 24-hour days with no sleep, eating, or drinking accounted for, just you and your smokes. How many full freaking days? I bet you always say I wish I had more time to get all things done that I need to or always wanted to. Please see why we aren't going to give them anymore time. Going forward I am not going to discuss the basic side effects in depth that are usually associated with smoking such as smell, taste, skin complexion because if you want that information there are so many other sources. You are not paying for that, you are paying to quit smoking, and you will tell smoking to fuck off. Your fucking got this.

I will provide some statistics I have found through my research because stats do work and these stats truthfully show how that bad your relationship with Puffy is for you. I am going to explain some of their stats into more simpler forms and laments terms. Here are some general smoking stats from Center for Disease Control website[1]. The overall mortality rate (chance of death) among both male and female smokers in the United States is about three times higher than that among similar people who never smoked. The major causes of increased chance of death among smokers are diseases that are related to smoking, including the big C cancer, respiratory (breathing) and vascular or in common terms heart disease. Did you know that Cigarette smoking causes about one of every five deaths in the United States each year? Now think about that number, 20 percent of all deaths are caused by smoking your faithful death sticks. Cigarette smoking including deaths from second-hand smoke is estimated to cause more than 480,000 deaths annually, of those 278,544 are most likely men while 201,773 are women. From my research and almost any other medical professionals smoking causes premature death, as life expectancy for smokers is at least 10 years shorter than for non-smokers. One great thing is that by quitting smoking before the age of 40 reduces the risk of dying from smoking-related disease by about 90%. 90 FUCKING PERCENT, fuck yeah. Hey Puffy Fuck Off, take your butt and get the fuck out of here.

---

[1] https://www.cdc.gov/tobacco/data_statistics/fact_sheets/adult_data/cig_smoking/index.htm

An interesting fact is that men are more likely to be current cigarette smokers than women. Nearly 16% of all men are smokers compared to about 12% for women. According to the CDC cigarette smoking is the leading cause of preventable disease and death in the United States. In 2017, an estimated 34.3 million adults in the United States currently smoked cigarettes. More than 16 million Americans live with a smoking-related disease. Thankfully with changes in society, culture and regulations smoking has declined from 20.9% (nearly 21 of every 100 adults) in 2005 to 14.0% (14 of every 100 adults) in 2017, and the proportion of ever smokers who have quit has increased. Join this stat and tell smoking, tell nicotine, tell the government and smoky to fuck off.

Let me ask you a simple question, what is lung cancer? Now stop and run all the science shit in your head and recite what to yourself know about cancer. Sit there like in your old school days or partial conversations you overheard since it will never happen to you anyway. Take the full 10 minutes to come up with your conclusion before presenting. Skip ahead if you feel you already know enough but please feel free to continue reading for more awesome science shit anyways. Now let's dive right into topic, and get right to the most common one and the one that hits home the most. The big C aka cancer. God bless just recently my mom was diagnosed with lung cancer. Thankfully she has had her operation, they removed 40% of one of her lungs and she is recovering. Mom finally quit and they say they should have gotten it before it spread further. The thing is she had been smoking for 40 years so really, she only has one person to blame. She is a fighter and I know we are lucky as we got more minutes to spend with her and she has more minutes to spend away from Smokey so please don't let yourself become the unlucky one.

According to the CDC, their definition is that Cancer[2] is a disease in which cells in the body grow out of control. In simple plain terms, it spreads through your body destroying everything in its path like a slow tsunami of death killing anything healthy in its path. When cancer starts in the lungs, it is called lung cancer. Lung cancer begins in the lungs and may spread to lymph nodes or other organs in the body, such as the brain. Cancer from other organs also may spread to the lungs. Now like I said above it spreads just killing anything it comes into path with.

Cancer is the second leading cause of death in the United States, only outdoing heart disease. One in every four deaths in the United States is due to cancer according to the American Cancer Society however lung cancer (both small cell and non-small cell) is the second most common cancer in both men and women (not counting skin cancer). In men, prostate cancer is more common, while in women breast cancer is more common. About 13% of all new cancers are lung cancers. The American Cancer Society's estimates for lung cancer in the United States for 2019 about 228,150 new cases of lung cancer (116,440 in men and 111,710 in women) and roughly 142,670 deaths from lung cancer (76,650 in men and 66,020 in women). Lung cancer is by far the leading cause of cancer death among both men and women. Each year, more people die of lung cancer than of colon, breast, and prostate cancers combined. Cancer is unfortunately usually a death sentence.

---

[2] https://gis.cdc.gov/Cancer/USCS/DataViz.html

In my opinion the biggest risk from smoking is lung cancer and as mentioned with my mom it's the most personal so here are some of signs and symptoms of lung cancer according to the CDC. Guess what most of the time lung cancers do not cause any symptoms until they have spread, but some people with early lung cancer do have symptoms. Luckily, we got to mom's just in time, 6 months later and it would have been a complexly different story. If you go to your doctor when you first notice symptoms, you might be diagnosed at an earlier stage, when treatment is more likely to be effective. Most of these symptoms are more likely to be caused by something other than lung cancer. Still, if you have any of these problems, it's important to see your doctor right away so the cause can be found and treated, if needed. The most common symptoms of lung cancer are a cough that does not go away or gets worse, coughing up blood or rust-colored sputum (spit or phlegm), chest pain, loss of appetite, shortness of breath, feeling weak, exhausted or tired, Infections such as bronchitis and pneumonia that don't go away or keep coming back. It is even worst if you leave the symptoms to long and the lung cancer spreads to other parts of the body, it may cause changes to your nervous system such as headache, weakness or numbness of an arm or leg, dizziness, balance problems, or seizures or from cancer spread to the brain, it can cause bone pains or yellowing of the skin and eyes (jaundice), from cancer spread to the liver , your lymph nodes may swell(collection of immune system cells) such as those in the neck or above the collarbone

If you happen to luck out and not get fucked by Cancer then you also have this bad boy to worry about. It is a lot less common but it's still that slimy fucker waiting in the corner just to stab you in the back, and that mother fucker is Emphysema. Well fuck Emphysema too.

Emphysema according to NCBI National Center for Biotechnology Information[3], which just happens an amazing source for information about medical knowledge. It is amazing what information is out there for anyone to see. Pulmonary emphysema, a progressive lung disease, is a form of chronic obstructive pulmonary disease (COPD). COPD is the third leading cause of death in the United States and fourth leading cause of the death worldwide. The World Health Organization (WHO) estimates suggest that it will rise to be the third most common cause of death worldwide by 2020. COPD includes patients with chronic bronchitis and emphysema. Emphysema is caused by chronic and significant exposure to noxious gases of which, death stick smoking remains the most common cause, and 80% to 90% of COPD patients are cigarette smokers identified, with 10% to 15% smokers developing COPD. However, in smokers, the symptoms also depend on the intensity of smoking, years of exposure, and baseline lung function. Symptoms usually begin after at least 20 pack per year of tobacco exposure and yes smart ass before you mention it. You can skip this if you want because it is going to sound techy.

---

[3] https://www.ncbi.nlm.nih.gov/books/NBK482217/

According to the NCBI[4], Biomass fuels and other environmental pollutants such as sulfur dioxide and particulate matter are recognized as an important cause in developing countries affecting women and children greatly. However, it only contributes to 1% to 2% cases of COPD. There is no known, definitive treatment which can modify Emphysema however, risk-factor modification and management of symptoms have been proven effective in slowing the disease progression and optimizing the quality of living which in laments terms means basically your fucked for life and there is no real treatment, too bad so sad, thank you for playing but just in case there are some things you can try to keep it in check. Now according to our friends in the land down under Australia, their government site[5], COPD affects 1 in 20 Australians over 45 years of age and is the fifth most common cause of death in Australia. People who smoke are more than 6 times as likely to have COPD as non-smokers. Even people who have given up are 5 times as likely to develop emphysema as people who have never smoked. For some more amazing statistics or writer fluff as I like to call it. According to the CDC[6] which states number of deaths from chronic lower respiratory diseases (including asthma) in the United States is approximately 160,201. Chronic lower respiratory diseases (including asthma) deaths per 100,000 population is around 49% it's cause of death rank is number 4. The number of bronchitis (chronic and unspecified) deaths was 502 while the number of emphysema deaths was 7,085 and finally the number of deaths from other chronic lower respiratory diseases (excluding asthma) was a whopping 149,050.

---

[4] https://www.ncbi.nlm.nih.gov/books/NBK482217/

[5] https://www.healthdirect.gov.au/emphysema-and-copd-statistics

[6] https://www.cdc.gov/tobacco/basic_information/health_effects/respiratory/index.htm

Finally, I could now start going on about heart disease for days or as the professionals call it vascular disease however it's too broad for us to be wasting a ton of time on it so just know it's really fucking bad for the ticker. No really google that shit because the point of this is not to educate but motivate you to tell cigarettes to fuck off. With this said we still need some filler to make our simple process look so much more in depth. Really once you read ahead you will think to yourself holy shit this is common sense so read to be enlightened by the topic. Once again according to our friends at the CDC fact number one is that both heart disease and stroke are cardiovascular (heart and blood vessel) diseases (CVDs). Heart disease[7] includes several types of heart conditions but the most common type in the United States is coronary heart disease (also known as coronary artery disease), which is narrowing (thinning) of the blood vessels that carry blood to the heart. This can cause chest pain, heart attack (when blood flow to the heart becomes blocked and a section of the heart muscle is damaged or dies), heart failure (when the heart cannot pump enough blood and oxygen to support other organs), Arrhythmia (when the heart beats irregularly).

---

[7]https:\www.cdc.gov\tobacco\basic_information\health_effects\heart_disease\index.htm

A stroke[8] occurs when the blood supply to the brain is blocked or when a blood vessel in the brain bursts, initiating brain tissue to die. Stroke can cause disability (such as paralysis, muscle weakness, trouble speaking, memory loss) or death. Now after reading all these facts one has to ask themselves, how Is smoking related to heart disease and stroke? Well to answer that question smoking is a major cause of cardiovascular disease and causes one of every four deaths from CVDs. Smoking can raise triglycerides (a type of fat in your blood), lower "good" cholesterol aka HDL, make blood sticky and more likely to clot, which can block blood flow to the heart and brain damage cells that line the blood vessels increase the buildup of plaque (fat, cholesterol, calcium, and other substances) in blood vessels cause thickening and narrowing of blood vessels

Finally, here are some stats according to my authorities above the border at Health Canada[9]. They say that the risk of coronary heart disease increases with both the number of years smoked and the number of cigarettes smoked per day. Even individuals who smoke fewer than 5 cigarettes per day are at an increased risk of this condition. There were 36,860 deaths from coronary heart disease in 2007. Research has shown that, in 2002, smoking was accountable for almost half of all deaths from coronary heart disease among Canadians under the age of 45 years. Smokers are up to 4 times more likely to have a sudden cardiac death than are non-smokers. People exposed to second-hand smoke[10] are also at increased risk of coronary heart disease. The good thing is the treatment of coronary heart disease aims to improve blood flow to the heart. Types of treatment include lifestyle changes such as smoking cessation and exercise, drug treatment, and interventions such as angioplasty or heart surgery.

---

[8]https:\www.cdc.gov\tobacco\basic_information\health_effects\heart_disease\index.htm

[9]https://www.canada.ca/en/health-canada/services/health-

Basically, the conclusion to all this information is it's telling us that smoking kills you, its roughly the same stats no matter where you go in the world. An interesting note is that not once during all this research did I find one advantage to smoking now because I couldn't find any good stuff about cigarettes here is some more boring shit but still scary but still boring shit according to the CDC. Exposure to second-hand smoke causes an estimated 41,000 deaths each year among adults in the United States it causes a further 7,333 annual deaths from lung cancer and causes 33,951 annual deaths from heart disease. Men who smoke increase their risk of dying from bronchitis and emphysema by 17 times; from cancer of the throat, lung, and bronchus by more than 23 times. Smoking increases the risk of dying from coronary heart disease among middle-aged men by almost four times. Women who smoke increase their risk of dying from bronchitis and emphysema by 12 times; from cancer of the trachea, lung, and bronchus by more than 12 times. Between 1960 and 1990, deaths from lung cancer among women increased by more than 500%. In 1987, lung cancer surpassed breast cancer to become the leading cause of cancer death among U.S. women. During 2010–2014, almost 282,000 women (56,359 women each year) will die from lung cancer. Smoking increases the risk of dying from coronary heart disease among middle-aged women by almost five times as mentioned in the very beginning of the chapter I could go on for days about the smell and moral implications but once again that is not the intent of this book. The only intent is to tell smoking to Fuck Off so let's get to it.

concerns/tobacco/legislation/tobacco-product-labelling/smoking-heart-disease.html

[10]https://www.canada.ca/en/health-canada/services/health-concerns/tobacco/legislation/tobacco-product-labelling/second-hand-smoke.html

Chapter 3 – Day 1 – Telling Puffy to Fuck Off

A new day is upon you with the main goal of today is to break your routine. Let's get the hugs and tugs out of the way and as always first of all; thank you for taking this first step to a smoke free life by telling smoking to fuck off, I wish you all the best. This will be one of the most difficult things you will ever do in your lifetime if not the most difficult thing since you are about to rewire your whole system from your brain to your body to your identity and even to your culture. I would wish you good luck but this journey has absolutely nothing to do with luck, these are the first steps of your personal journey to kick the dirty habit and every single choice is resting on your shoulders. Every excuse, every whine and complaint are on you. There are no risks or chances, you control every single decision. You have 100% control over the results. An important thing to remember is that this journey has everything to do with change, it will give you the power to make a new you, a healthier, sexier and more financially independent you. So finally, after all my fluff we are advancing. Let's get started.

The very first thing we need to do is break routine because 50% of smoking is habit not addiction. We blame the addiction but we like the habit. Think about that how many times have you been outside sitting, its 1:30 in the afternoon so you have a much-needed smoke, then 15 mins you are bored and you want to have another one. Then you realize and say no, I have to wait these are expensive so I now have to wait about an hour before I can have another and then 20 minutes later you get the craving and have another, now it is 2:30 and you reward yourself with that smoke. Guess what? Now you have technically smoked 2 cigarettes in an hour. Hello Einstein guess what happens in about 20 minutes when you are board. Wash, rinse, repeat. A major obstacle I found is this, we as humans tend to follow the same routines every day and look for the paths of least resistance. It is simple human nature, it is the same routine each day, day in and day out. Smokers don't worry about these habits or routines because they are being driven by addiction. All you are really thinking about is that next ciggy. You know it's true. Don't smoke for 2 hours then tell me your first thought. Exactly addiction.

Let's get one thing straight as well, you are not the victim, nobody did this to you but yourself sunshine so get that mentality out of your head. Because if you don't you will fail over and over again. Own up to your past failures, by your own accord you made each decision of your own freewill. I know personally when I started smoking, not one single person forced me to, no one held me down. I choose of my own freewill to take that cigarette and subsequently the first puff. I am correct in saying that I was very young and uneducated about the issue in the beginning but it was still me who started this vicious cycle and so it gets left to me alone to break it. As I said in your defense you were probably not properly educated at that time as well especially if you were born prior to 1990. Up to around 1995 smoking was still cool, it was relaxing and it was the thing to do, it was cheap and readily available, at that time we knew the problems and health issues that smoking caused but we didn't care. In the end it was you put who put that cancer stick in your mouth. So just own it and so you can change It. You and only you are responsible for your own outcome.

Now let's get ready to start our day. The night before judgement day. Please smoke as much as you want. Smoke as many as you want. Smoke the whole pack if you want to but remember you are having your very last smoke, go ahead and enjoy it. Be the little train that could, puff, puff, puff, choo, choo. Savor the taste, love the smell, feel the rush and embrace the afterglow. Make this smoke sexy, make it sensual, think of it like breaking up from a long-time partner and you get have that goodbye sex. It's amazing sex because you know it's the last time you will get this feeling, you are not ever going to feel this again. It's now time to the smokes pack it up and move on elsewhere. Sad joke but I couldn't refuse. Enjoy every thrust to your lips, savor our every moist drop of nicotine as it soaks into your tongue. The last time their tip will enter your mouth. This is your last taste because you are leaving that sexy beast, Puffy McPufferson and moving forward with your life. After you butt out Puffy and say your final goodbyes, explain to them why this just isn't working anymore and why smoking is a piece of shit habit and can sincerely from the deepest recesses of my heart fuck off.

The night before judgement day you will need to set your alarm clock so that you wake up early. This is an absolute must do because your alarm clock change fluctuates the morning from normal day. Only 10 minutes will work, you can take longer if you want but for this today's purpose it's a very important part. The goal is you are breaking the daily routine. You are also sub-concisely telling yourself that you are willing to give up 10 minutes of sleeping, I know most people like my wife cherish every minute of sleep. It is as valuable to her as my smokes were to me. Now even if you do get up or have a smoke right away you fail today's task and skip the whole process for the day, I mean if you can't even fight the battle of giving up 10 minutes of sleep. How are you going to resist old Puffy? Remember the most important footstep is to not be a pussy, don't be weak. You don't realize this but you are stronger than you ever imagined. You have to fight the urge to fail. You have to fight every excuse you create and no matter what happens do not bend and do not have that smoke. If you have to run away and cry then please do it, no one will judge you. Know that every single piece of your success is simply based upon being strong and not giving in to your urges by having just one puff because remember even that puff means you are still smoking's bitch. The number one reason for failing to quit smoking is keeping that crutch, that safety net of having just one. Let me ask you this smart one, how can you quit if you keep having just one?

Close your eyes and think about your routine. As most it probably goes like this. You wake up and have a smoke right away. Depending on your circumstance it might be right in bed or like myself would have to get dressed and go outside in the rain or cold. Either way you're smart and you get the picture and if this is what you do or no matter what type of schedule you have such as, wake up make coffee, smoke then smoke again. Some people are so addicted they literally think I went 6 hours without smoking and need to make up for it. I know if you are like my dad, he wakes up in the middle of the night to have one. But back to our day, now we rush to the bathroom you use the toilet, shower, and get ready. From there we know the rest of that story. You will notice I don't really finish the whole story because there is no need to waste any further time here as we only have so many minutes remaining in our bank account.

You are going to wake up 10 minutes early and not have a cigarette, one single smoke nor puff for the whole day. You are going to lay in bed and just think to yourself how today is a new day and today you are going forward with a new you. Think of all the good things that are going to happen to your life, it's ok to lay here and daydream. Repeat to yourself and just say no each time you get a craving; I know it sounds easy but it's going to suck. You know it and so do I but guess what, did you realize you are already smoke free? You have been smoke free since you went to bed the night before. Go ahead what take whatever time you went to bed say it is 11PM and if you woke up at 6:50AM, figure out the time difference. It is 7 hours and 50 minutes smoke free or 470 minutes. After waiting out the 10 mins extra guess what you are now 480 minutes smoke free. Now are you dying, has the world come crashing down on you, have you split the very fabric of time and space. No instead now you are a little edgy and a bit anxious, a little groggy and things don't quite seem right but guess what, things are not right because you have completed a task you have not concisely done in years. You have managed to wake up and skip your smoke; you broke your routine and now you have 480 minutes smoke free.

When was the last time you were 8 hours smoke free? You already have the head start, there is no hour one, hour one is already done. You are already on hour 8. Remember a smoke is going to take about 2 minutes of your time. When you smoke you are going to sit there for a solid two minutes and fill your body with poisonous chemicals and gain nothing but temporary relief from pain that you are going to experience every single time you try to quit. Now normally you would cave but not today. You already have 480 minutes in are you going to throw everything away for 2-minute quickie. You are willing to throw away for 480 minutes of success for 2 minutes of failure. Just keep remembering how many minutes you are throwing away every time you want to sneak Puffy back into your life. They don't care about you they are always there to hold you back. Always there to let you fail. Good old Puffy. Now that you are on minute number 485 because your first craving has taken you about 5 minutes to pass. It's time to go ahead with your day. There is nothing special, no rules, no further steps just be a decent person and don't harm anyone either physically, verbally or mentally, remember that nicotine only takes about 3 days to detox from your system so it will get better. Just keep track of your smoke free minutes and realize that 2 mins compared to how many you are at is just not worth it. No matter what you do, do not even cave for a puff because a single puff is failure and in saying so here are some tips to help you.

Chapter 4 Tips for Quitting – The Weapons to Fucking Off

Once again as we have discussed numerous times that quitting smoking is the hardest thing you will ever do but its all on you and rests solely on your shoulders. It's a lot of weight but you can do it so let's talk about why quitting is so hard. We all know the health risks of smoking as mentioned in Chapter 2, but that doesn't make it any easier to kick the habit. According to our friends at Helpguide.org[11], it doesn't matter if you're an occasional smoker or a lifetime pack-a-day smoker, quitting is really tough. Smoking tobacco is both a physical addiction[12] (your body)and a psychological habit (your mind). The nicotine from cigarettes provides a momentary and addictive high (dopamine). Eliminating that regular hit of nicotine causes your body to experience physical withdrawal symptoms and cravings. Because of nicotine's "feel good" effect on the brain, you may turn to cigarettes as a fast and reliable way to boost your outlook, relieve stress, and unwind. Smoking can also be a coping mechanism for depression, anxiety, or even boredom. Quitting means finding different, healthier ways to cope with those feelings.

---

[11] https://www.helpguide.org/articles/addictions/how-to-quit-smoking.htm

[12] https://www.helpguide.org/harvard/how-addiction-hijacks-the-brain.htm

As mentioned, in chapter 3 smoking is also ingrained as a daily ritual, it is part of your very existence. I mean who are you without your cigarette. Smoking may be an automatic response for you to smoke a cigarette with your morning coffee, while taking a break at work or school, or on your commute home at the end of a frantic day. Or maybe your friends, family, or co-workers smoke, and it's become part of the way you relate with them, as gloomy as it sounds it becomes a bond amongst other smokers. Don't you find it so much easier to make random conversation with a stranger if they are smoking. To successfully quit smoking, you'll need to address both the addiction and the habits. The routines that go along with it. But don't worry it can be done. With this book, the right plan and the proper support system then any smoker can kick the addiction no matter if you've tried and failed multiple times before. Every time the clock can start over. Now let's talk about that plan. Even though some smokers quit by going through the ever so dreaded cold turkey method but in general most people do better with a custom-made plan to keep themselves on track. Do not feel bad if you can't go cold turkey and need to use a cessation product, I am the first to admit that I used nicotine gum myself when I successfully quit. This is going to be a battle and any weapons in your arsenal can only help the cause as long as you are not replacing one for the other. Remember you will need to eventually quit the cessation product too if you are substituting one for another. There are a ton of good cessation products on the market my personal favorite was Nicorette. However, a good quit plan addresses both the short-term challenge of stopping smoking and the long-term challenge of preventing relapse or climbing back in bed with Puffy. It should also be personalized to your specific needs and your smoking habits. Your body and mind are no one else's houses, this is a one-person game.

Here are some questions to ask yourself. Take the time to contemplate of what kind of smoker you are, which instants of your life call for a cigarette, and why. This will aid you to identify which tips, techniques, or therapies may be most advantageous for you. Ask yourself am I a heavy smoker (more than a pack a day)? Or are you more of a social smoker (only when around friends or drinking)? Would a nicotine patch do the job? Are there certain activities, places, or people you associate with smoking? Do you feel the necessity to smoke after every meal or whenever you break for coffee? Do you reach for cigarettes when you're feeling stressed or down? Or is your cigarette smoking linked to other addictions, such as alcohol or gambling? Think to yourself if you can Identify your smoking triggers.

One of the greatest things you can do to help yourself quit is to recognize the things that make you want to smoke, including specific circumstances, events, feelings, and people. Lots of people do it and if it works go for it, they keep a craving journal because it helps them you zone in on your patterns and triggers. For a week or so leading up to your quit date, keep a log of your smoking. Note the moments in each day when you crave a cigarette:

- What time was it?
- How intense was the craving (on a scale of 1-10)?
- What were you doing?
- Who were you with?
- How were you feeling?
- How did you feel after smoking?

Another trigger question is do I smoke to dismiss unpleasant feelings? Many people smoke to manage unpleasant feelings such as stress, depression, loneliness, and anxiety. When you have a bad day, it can seem like cigarettes are your only friend, good old Puffy. As much comfort as cigarettes provide, though, it's important to remember that there are healthier and more effective ways to keep your shitty feelings in check. These may include exercising, meditating, relaxation strategies[13], or simple breathing exercises. For many people, an important aspect of giving up smoking is to find other ways to handle these difficult feelings[14] without whirling back to cigarettes. Even when cigarettes are no longer a part of your life, the painful and unpleasant feelings that may have provoked you to smoke in the past will still continue. So, it's worth spending some time thinking about the different ways you intend to deal with stressful situations and the daily irritations that would normally have you lighting up.

---

[13]https://www.helpguide.org/articles/stress/relaxation-techniques-for-stress-relief.htm

[14]https://www.helpguide.org/articles/mental-health/emotional-intelligence-toolkit.htm

Tips for evading common triggers. Many people smoke when they drink, they go hand in hand. Try switching to non-alcoholic drinks or drink only in places where smoking inside is prohibited. Alternatively, try snacking on nuts or ice, chewing on a cocktail stick or sucking on a straw. Here is another nasty trigger. Other smokers. When friends, family, and co-workers smoke around you, it can be twice as difficult to give up or avoid relapse. In your workplace, find non-smokers to have your breaks with or find other things to do, such as taking a walk or reading a book. End of a meal can be a fucking nightmare for most smokers. For some smokers, ending a meal means lighting up, and the prospect of giving that up may seem frightening. I considered my dessert to be cigarettes and this was my hardest one to give up because I eat all the time. However, you can try replacing that moment after a meal with something else, such as a sweet, dessert, or a stick of gum. I replaced my after-meal smokes with nicotine gum but soon I found myself getting addicted to the gum as well.

Once you tell Puffy to fuck off, you'll likely experience a number of physical symptoms as your body withdraws from nicotine. Nicotine withdrawal begins swiftly, usually starting within an hour of the last cigarette and peaking two to three days later. Withdrawal symptoms can last for a few days to several weeks and differ from person to person. Just to let you know its been a full 2 years and still every day I have to remind myself if throwing away a million minutes is worth two minutes of false satisfaction. Sometimes you just get triggered but remember triggers are out of your control and you give zero fucks to anything out of your control.

Common nicotine withdrawal symptoms include cigarette cravings, irritability, frustration, or anger, anxiety or nervousness. It can also cause difficulty concentrating, restlessness, increased appetite headaches, tremors (not the worm type), increased coughing and the list goes on forever. No matter what though unkind as these withdrawal symptoms may be, it's important to remember that they are only temporary. They will get better in a few weeks as the toxins are flushed from your body. In the meantime, let your friends and family know that you won't be your usual self and ask for their understanding. Remember it only takes roughly 72 hours to detox the nicotine.

While avoiding smoking triggers will help reduce your urge to smoke, you probably can't avoid cigarette cravings entirely. Fortunately, hungers don't last long—typically, about 5 or 10 minutes. If you're drawn to light up, remind yourself that the craving will soon pass and try to wait it out. It helps to be organized in advance by having strategies to deal with cravings. You must **distract yourself.** Do the dishes/clean as I found this worked wonders for me plus it gives the added satisfaction of a clean home. A clean home provides one of the most positive environments. Another great distraction is to find a fidget. I used a poker chip. I don't gamble but it worked perfect. It was small, had zero value just the perfect size to be able to play with it in my pocket, it become symbol of new me. It was my bank to hold my new currency. When my hands needed occupation, it gave me something to fidget with. You can exercise, take a shower, or call a friend because human interaction will help in the end. The activity doesn't matter as long as it gets your mind off smoking. Remind yourself why you quit. Focus on your reasons for quitting, including the health benefits (lowering your risk for heart disease and lung cancer, for example), improved appearance, money you're saving, and enhanced self-esteem. Get out of a tempting situation. Where you are or what you're doing may be triggering the craving. What is making you think about Puffy? Whenever you triumph over a hunger, give yourself a reward to keep yourself inspired.

There are many varied methods that have effectively helped people to kick the smoking routine. While you may be successful with the first method you try, more likely you'll have to try a number of different methods or a combination of treatments to find the ones that work best for you. There are many medications for which I have tried them all. There are smoking cessation medications can ease withdrawal symptoms and reduce cravings. They are most effective when used as part of a complete stop smoking program monitored by your physician. Talk to your doctor about your options and whether an anti-smoking medication is right for you. There is also nicotine replacement therapy which involves "replacing" cigarettes with other nicotine substitutes, such as nicotine gum, patch, lozenge, inhaler, or nasal spray. It relieves some of the withdrawal symptoms by delivering small and steady doses of nicotine into your body without the tars and poisonous gases found in cigarettes. This type of treatment helps you focus on breaking your psychological addiction and makes it easier to concentrate on learning new behaviors and coping skills. If you do not like the nicotine option then there are **non-nicotine medication options.** These medications help you stop smoking by reducing cravings and withdrawal symptoms without the use of nicotine. Medications such as bupropion (Zyban) and varenicline (Chempax) are intended for short-term use only.

Finally, there are many other therapies such as **hypnosis**. This is a popular option that has produced excellent results for many smokers struggling to resign from a life of nicotine; hypnosis can work by getting you into a deeply relaxed state where you are open to suggestions that strengthen your resolve to stop smoking and increase your negative feelings toward cigarettes. I must admit that I never tried this because I have mixed feelings on hypnosis. Some try
acupuncture which just happens to be one of the oldest known medical techniques, acupuncture is thought to work by triggering the release of endorphins (natural pain relievers) that allow the body to relax. As a smoking cessation aid, acupuncture can be helpful in handling smoking withdrawal symptoms.

Others have tried behavioral therapy which focuses on the habitual behaviors or rituals involved in smoking. Behavior therapy focuses on learning new coping skills and breaking those habits. Lastly there are the motivational therapies such as self-help books like this one and websites can provide a number of ways to motivate yourself to give up smoking. One well known example is calculating the monetary savings. Some people have been able to find the motivation to quit just by calculating how much money they will save.

Now one asks what happens what to do if you slip or relapse, most people try to stop smoking several times before they kick the habit for good, so don't beat yourself up if you slip up and smoke a cigarette. Instead, turn the relapse into a rebound by learning from your mistake. Analyze what happened right before you started smoking again, identify the triggers or trouble spots you ran into, and make a new stop-smoking plan that eliminates them. It's also important to emphasize the difference between a slip and a relapse. If you start smoking again, it doesn't mean that you can't get back on the plane. You can choose to learn from the slip and let it motivate you to try harder or you can use it as an excuse to go back to your smoking habit. But the choice is yours. A slip doesn't have to turn into a full-blown relapse. You're not a failure if you slip up. It doesn't mean you can't quit for good. Whatever you do, don't let a slip become a rabbit hole.

Throw out the rest of the pack or smoke them all up the night before Judgment Day. It's important to get back on the non-smoking track as soon as possible. Discover the trigger. Exactly what was it that made you smoke again? Decide how you will manage with that issue the next time it comes up. Learn from your experience. What has been most helpful? What didn't work? Are you using a medicine to help you quit? Call your doctor if you start smoking again. Some medicines cannot be used if you're smoking at the same time.

Finally ask yourself how can quitting smoking be helpful?[15]
Now that you know how smoking can be harmful to your
health and the health of those around you, here are some
ways quitting can be accommodating. If you quit smoking,
you will extend your life, diminish your risk of disease
(including heart disease, heart attack, high blood
pressure, lung cancer[16], throat cancer, emphysema,
ulcers, gum disease, and other conditions), you will feel
healthier. After quitting, you won't cough[17] as much, you'll
have fewer sore throats and you will increase your stamina,
look better. Quitting can help you prevent face wrinkles[18], get
rid of tarnished teeth, and improve your skin. Expand your
sense of taste and smell. Who knew boiled potatoes tasted so
damn good, seriously wait for the flavors to return. A favorite
of mine is that you will finally save some of your hard-earned
money.
The people at Verywellmind.com[19] point out the benefits
always far outweigh the work it takes to quit
smoking. The sense of inner strength and belief in our ability
to accomplish challenging goals grows immeasurably.
Quitting tobacco for most people represents an out of reach
dream we've carried with us for many years. Learning that we
are indeed strong enough and worthy a life free of
addiction opens doors long closed. Ex-smokers often take on a
sport they always wanted to do, change course in their
careers, or go back to school.

---

[15] https://www.medicinenet.com/smoking_and_heart_disease/article.htm#how_can_quitting_smoking_be_helpful

[16] https://www.medicinenet.com/lung_cancer_pictures_slideshow/article.htm

[17] https://www.medicinenet.com/chronic_cough/article.htm

[18] https://www.medicinenet.com/wrinkles/article.htm

[19] https://www.verywellmind.com/nicotine-use-4157297

Smoking cessation is a life-changer.[20] You'll see. The odds are against you if you don't quit. If you are a lifetime smoker, your risk of dying a tobacco-related death is about 50 percent. Additionally, on average, lifetime smokers lose 10 years of life over those who don't smoke. Recall 480,000 lives are lost to tobacco in the United States every year, and six million die of tobacco-related deaths worldwide annually, However, if you quit smoking before your 40th birthday, you'll reduce your risk of dying from a smoking-related disease by 90 percent. Fewer people are smoking today in the U.S. than ever before. In 2005, 21 out of every 100 people over the age of 18 (20.9 percent) smoked in the United States. By 2014, that number had dropped to 17 per 100 adults (16.8 percent/40 million smokers), and continues to go down.

[20]   https://www.verywellmind.com/quit-smoking-benefits-between-one-and-nine-months-2824386

We can thank aggressive anti-smoking legislation and campaigns for pushing American smokers in the right direction. They've educated us about the dangers associated with tobacco use, but in countries without this benefit, smoking rates are much higher. There are one billion smokers around the world today. Eighty percent of them live in low- and middle-income countries. Quitting smoking isn't as difficult as you think. Yes, it takes work and yes, it takes some time[21]. That said, the hard part happens early on, and with some education about what's ahead[22] and the support to get through it, you'll be pleasantly surprised that recovery from nicotine addiction is doable and a finite task. You won't always miss smoking, there will be cravings but you won't miss smoking itself. You will miss the nicotine[23]. Every smoker is afraid to quit smoking. Nicotine addiction[24] forces us to continue smoking long after we want to stop. We think about quitting daily, but then the fear of letting go sets in and we put it off. The fact is, no matter when you quit, you'll feel that fear every smoker is familiar with. Push through it and move forward. Your anxiety will diffuse with a little time.

---

21   https://www.verywellmind.com/why-the-first-year-of-smoking-cessation-is-so-important-2824682

22 https://www.verywellmind.com/surviving-nicotine-withdrawal-2824750

23 https://www.verywellmind.com/will-i-miss-smoking-forever-2824756

24 https://www.verywellmind.com/nicotine-addiction-101-2825018

Chapter 5 - Day 2 Repeat the Worst Day of Your Life

Day 2 is relatively simple, sarcasm noted. Let's get right to it and let you know way to fucking go you made it through the first 24 hours. I am so proud of you. You ignored Puffy's calls and texts. You officially have 24 hours in with no cigarettes, that is 1440 minutes. If you are honest to yourself, you did not cheat, you did not even have just that one puff then you have done something amazing. It is a wonder because the miracle you performed was something you have been telling yourself was impossible and something you not done since you started smoking. Repeat the phenomenon to yourself that this is the first time in so many years that I have gone 24 hours completely smoke free. You got 24 hours into the bank. Remember that credits can quickly balance out all those debits.

If you cheated that's okay as it just means you did well yesterday. You only had so many puffs or only one smoke which you should be happy about but you need to start from Day One again today. If you haven't been able to go the full 24 hours without having a puff even just one puff off a friend or a cigarette butt since you know you smoked your last smoke 2 nights ago. That one puff alone means you are losing the Power of the 24. However, if you were honest to yourself because the only person you would be lying to is yourself then please proceed the challenge of day 2. This is your game and you are the only player. The ball is in your court. I want you to now close your eyes and think about how fucking bad yesterday was. Think of all the shit you went through all the breakdowns, cold sweats, freak-outs, anxiety and just general shitty feelingless. The pain and the suffering you experienced is well worth it and remember to own your whole 24 fucking hours. Now here we go with day 2.

Step 1: Wake up and do not kill people, repeat the following statement three times, I shall kill no mother fucker that pisses me off today. Then repeat smoking fuck off three times. At your best today try to keep talking to a minimum, whenever possible avoid people and family members, especially your family members because they are the only ones cheering for you. They are like your cheerleaders and you wouldn't bring them into the big game. This is your game; this is on you, but it's the healthier you, the winner in the mirror, the new you. You are the hero of this fucking story; you are writing the legacy so what are you going to do? Are you going to cough and sputter like the old broken-down Kia Soul or are you going to live a new vibrant revamped life like the good old punch buggy?

You are going to take on any support your friends and family give you. You will receive and be grateful for every good job you hear from them. You know what if you need self-reassurance then you will surely get a good job from them and a pat on the back. When you do have to be around them try to be nice and replace fuck off with no problem. Remember always apologize if you are wrong. By this point you have woken up and your feet hit the floor. You went through your little mantra, prayer or whatever it is called now whatever you do, do not have that cigarette. No matter what urge or any other pain you must suffer do not give in. That death stick is going to bring a simple two minutes pleasure and for what a little stress, a little anxiety. What are you a little bitch? To be blunt are you are wimp? Realize you are going to throw away 24 hours of being smoke free. 24 Hours of suffering through the worst day of your life for what maybe two minutes. Let me ask you this are you stupid?

You have done the supposed impossible. You are throwing away 24 Hours at 60 Minutes equaling 1440 minutes of Hell. The Hell for two minutes of killing yourself. Why because someone was mean or you got cut off or you are worried? Really you are an adult, all of these are basic human interactions and feelings. You will never be able to avoid interactions or feelings. You must own them and handle them. The more I think about it, in the end all you are saying to yourself is I am willing to abandon 1438 Hell for two minutes of Heaven, if this was sex than maybe one would think about that deal but that's a different book.

Now go through your day and repeat hell again, if you have them take a sick day or vacation day then go for it. Technically you are sick and technically you are on a vacation to Hell. You must separate yourself from your triggers and then get to day 3. Day 3 will be easier. If you need to run around telling everybody how long it has been since your last puff then go ahead get your pat on the back because it will only service your ego. Now we are moving onward because that won't truly help you because we know deep down only your will power can get the job done. However positive reinforcement and encouragement doesn't hurt either. Remember this is a mind game, a true test of power. The withdrawal will hurt so bad it feels like a Saw movie. Just play the game and no matter happens keep fighting through. Fight through with all the fuck yous in the world and please battle through your day you go to bed. Just make it through the morning to night no matter what without a single puff. You are toughing than you think. You have a new bank balance full of minutes are you going to empty it for two whole minutes fake satisfaction. If you can name one true benefit you are getting then go ahead but its still an excuse. I bet you that if you wait five more minutes the feelings and pain will pass because in all honesty, we know it always will. Yes, it will eventually creep back but wash, rinse, repeat and just wait five more minutes. You are a smart person you get the fucking picture don't you.

Chapter 6 Day 3 Wash, Rinse, and Repeat

Remember Day 2 and all the stuff I told you well repeat and but now there is one big difference one gigantic accomplishment, you have officially gone two full days, 48 hours or most importantly now you have gone 2880 minutes without a smoke. You have completed the impossible twice now. You are a superstar. Almost reaching super hero status. Keep up the fantastic work. You should be so proud of yourself. Nobody else did it. You did it all on your own. You have now as a secondary bonus created a new routine for the first time in X amount of years smoking. You now have already woke up twice and done something difference than the status quo. Now let me ask you this, are you going to be an idiot and throw away the new you? When you speak of the new life you are building will you throw it all in the trash for a two-minute quickie Puffy? Even just a chat is flirting with destruction. Are you going to go back to your old habits? The answers to these questions are always going to be no because you are an adult and as a conscious grown-up you are responsible for your own choices. You have the ability to be anyone you want to be, you are creating your own world, your own reality and at any moment you can change them. You also control your own reality not Puffy.

Puffy might sneak back and might whisper all those sweet words, they really know how to hit all your buttons. They will try to remind you about all the times they have there for you, through rain or shine, flood or accident, and sickness or death. Here is a fact for you. The new you, INSERT YOU NAME has 48 hours of being smoke free. Unless you are a complete idiot nothing should ever come between you and your first million, now it could be dollars or minutes either way by not smoking you are only adding more of those to your future.

Now you are probably sitting here thinking to yourself wow this was a short chapter. Is this book missing something? My answer is no, because after paying this money it simply comes down to willpower and looking at the simple numbers. It is always up to you to say no, that's it, it is simply going minute to minute each day. There will always be nay sayers or other smokers who try to push back to their dark world then just fight back and push them fuckers away. Tell them all to fuck off. Remember they would quit if they could but they can't because they also are addicted. Now sit down and think about this one, the cigarette manufacturers could dip their cigarettes in shit and still be profitable. Now guess what if they all did it and all cigarettes were shit flavored nationwide you would still smoke them and you know why.

Continue going forward this process will be easier and easier every day. You now have 4320 minutes in your bank. Are you going to empty that account for a one to 2-minute smoke? If you feel the desire to puff just think about these following questions. Are you going to throw the effort away because you can't let go of your past? Do you fear personal growth? So are you chucking in the trash all the tears, pain and agony of going 4000 minutes without a smoke for what a 2-minute crutch? Are you that much of a pussy? Do you have no will power? You know it will not help in any true way by reconnecting with Puffy. Keep ignoring those pokes and little messages they send. Don't throw it away, because you were stressed or upset or any other excuse you find. Say to yourself who is it benefiting and do you have the will power? Wait 2 minutes without caving to the smoke, after 5 minutes then the emotions will have usually passed anyway.

Chapter 7 Day 4 Fuck Off Smoking for Good

As you will see telling cigarettes to fuck off isn't rocket science, numbers don't lie and once you see the number of minutes you are smoke free you will see why that smoking is no longer needed in your life. Remember all you have to do is keep reiterating to yourself day in and day out until one day you won't wake up and think about the sweet taste of smoke. To be honest you probably will still wake up with that feeling but on the bonus side you will wake up energized, refreshed and awake to the possibilities you didn't know once existed. Remember, Day 2 little mantra and all the stuff I told you and repeat such as, I shall kill no mother fucker that pisses me off today. I found this one worked best for me but I am sure if this doesn't work for you then you can create a new one.

The amazing thing about this quit smoking process is when you finally realize how many minutes of healthiness and happiness you are throwing away for 2 minutes when you have a cancer creator. Every day you will yearn for them but remember 2 minutes. Now go ahead and try going smoke free for 7 days, not even a puff. If you can't make a full one of 7 days because something happened and you didn't have the will power. We are human and things happen but an interesting conclusion I have drawn about smokers. My conclusion is that most smokers do quit however, they end up quitting trying to quit. All I can say to that mentality is what the fuck? In closing this chapter now have 5700 minutes in your book, how are you going to play the game? Can you reach 1 million minutes? I just did so come on and join the revolution.

Chapter 8 Horror Stories

I am going to share a few that have inspired me around the internet. My first story is **Roses**[25] story from the CDC website. I first must say oh my god Rose's story, it really hit home, because of my mother's recent battle with that miserable fucker, Cancer. Rose developed lung cancer from smoking cigarettes and showed great strength during nearly 2 years of intense treatments. She had chemotherapy, surgery, radiation, and a painful drainage tube in her chest. Doctors were able to remove the part of Rose's lung where the cancer had grown, but complications kept her in the hospital for a month with a chest tube. "The whole time it was in there, it was painful," she said. "The last 3 or 4 days, I literally cried." Finally, the chest tube came out—with a sharp, jabbing pain.

The cause of Rose's cancer—cigarettes—went back to her childhood. Rose started smoking at age 13 and continued for many years, smoking two packs a day. When she was 58 years old, her addiction to cigarettes nearly caused her to lose a foot because of clogged blood vessels. It was during that time she learned that she had lung cancer. "I regret picking up smoking in the first place," said Rose. "It's just addictive." Rose needed a second surgery after her lung cancer spread to her brain. She hoped that sharing the pain of her treatments would inspire other people to quit smoking as soon as possible. Rose wished that she had more days to spend with her friends and family—especially her three grandchildren, who meant the world to her. She died in January 2015, at age 60 from cancer caused by smoking.

[25] **https://www.cdc.gov/tobacco/campaign/tips/stories/rose.html**

Julia's[26] story hits two reasons, the first being my biggest fear is colon cancer, in my opinion one of the worst and here I am increasing the chances. I also chose this story for my daughter's name. Julia comes from a large and loving Mississippi family who came to her aid when she nearly died at age 49. Julia smoked for more than 20 years and developed colon cancer, which is a danger for all smokers. When her symptoms first started—cramps, diarrhea, and vomiting—she was puzzled and tried to manage them on her own. Then one day, the pain and bloating got much, much worse. A colon exam revealed that her intestines were completely blocked, which can be life threatening.

"I will never forget that day. I was so sick. They found the tumor in my colon and rushed me to the hospital," said Julia. She had surgery and then months of chemotherapy to treat the cancer. She needed an ostomy bag taped to a hole in her abdomen to collect waste. Julia's family took care of her and her young son, who was terrified to see his mother so sick. "The sickness really opened my eyes," said Julia. "By smoking, I was damaging myself and the people around me. I'm so glad I quit!"

Rebecca[27] is my youngest daughter's name and obviously it hits at tone. This story mirrored my childhood only I started smoking when I was in Grade 5. Rebecca is 53 years old but started smoking cigarettes at age 16. All of her family members smoked, and once she started smoking, she was hooked. Rebecca kept smoking into adulthood and tried to stop but soon discovered she had trouble quitting.

---

[26] https://www.cdc.gov/tobacco/campaign/tips/stories/julia.html

[27] https://www.cdc.gov/tobacco/campaign/tips/stories/rebecca.html

At age 33, Rebecca was diagnosed with depression. She smoked frequently when she felt depressed because she thought smoking might help her cope with her feelings. Rebecca felt ashamed when she smoked, so when she tried to quit and couldn't, she felt even more depressed. "That was just a vicious, vicious cycle," she said. To break the cycle, Rebecca knew she had to get care for her depression and quit smoking for good. Rebecca also lost some teeth as a result of gum disease, which can be caused by smoking. This further strengthened her resolve to lead a healthy lifestyle. Rebecca finally quit smoking, and she feels better — both mentally and physically. Rebecca is proud of her accomplishment. "It's about taking control and knowing where you want to be in your life.

Chapter 9 Closing Words – Hey Puffy Fuck Off

Now that we have made it through, I say congratulations on the new you. I am proud of you, so are your family and friends but most importantly you should be the proudest of yourself. Remember none of us fuckers did this for you. We have done nothing. None of us had to sweat, be anxious, not sleep or go through the depression. Remember you did though and you survived. With those kind parting words I must now say go out to this big beautiful world. Enjoy your life, embrace your change and use your willpower to take it every minute at a time. It will always be a battle as it is an addiction but as time goes on addiction fades as long as you don't feed it or stoke the fires.

The end game is to never put old dirty Puffy into your mouth. Remember to keep telling cigarettes to fuck off, tell Puffy to find someone else to fuck and keep collecting those minutes. I have over 1 million and counting. Once again that 2 years. Write me an email anytime to let me know your progress and give feedback of how this worked for you. If this book didn't work then great job still, just keep trying. Find what works for you as you must use one that works for you but it never hurts in trying to use my book again because if you had any will power at all then you won't need to. Yeah. Like I said in the beginning this is different kind of quit smoking book this isn't about sunshine and rainbows this is about quitting. Thank you again and so long, it has been an absolute pleasure working with you.

References

- https://www.ncbi.nlm.nih.gov/books/NBK482217/
- https://www.healthdirect.gov.au/emphysema-and-copd-statistics
- https://www.cdc.gov/tobacco/campaign/tips/stories/rebecca.html
- https://www.cdc.gov/tobacco/campaign/tips/stories/julia.html
- https://www.cdc.gov/tobacco/campaign/tips/stories/rose.html
- https://www.helpguide.org/articles/addictions/how-to-quit-smoking.htm
- https://www.canada.ca/en/health-canada/services/health-concerns/tobacco/legislation/tobacco-product-labelling/smoking-heart-disease.html
- https://www.cdc.gov/tobacco/basic_information/health_effects/heart_disease/index.htm
- https://www.verywellmind.com/nicotine-addiction-101-2825018
- https://www.verywellmind.com/will-i-miss-smoking-forever-2824756
- https://www.verywellmind.com/nicotine-use-4157297
- https://www.verywellmind.com/why-the-first-year-of-smoking-cessation-is-so-important-2824682
- https://www.verywellmind.com/surviving-nicotine-withdrawal-2824750

- https://www.verywellmind.com/nicotine-use-4157297

- https://www.verywellmind.com/quit-smoking-benefits-between-one-and-nine-months-2824386
- https://www.medicinenet.com/smoking_and_heart_disease/article.htm#how_can_quitting_smoking_be_helpful
- https://www.medicinenet.com/lung_cancer_pictures_slideshow/article.htm

- https://www.medicinenet.com/chronic_cough/article.htm

- https://www.medicinenet.com/wrinkles/article.htm

- https://www.canada.ca/en/health-canada/services/health-concerns/tobacco/legislation/tobacco-product-labelling/second-hand-smoke.html

- https://www.helpguide.org/articles/stress/relaxation-techniques-for-stress-relief.htm
- https://www.helpguide.org/articles/mental-health/emotional-intelligence-toolkit.htm
- https://www.helpguide.org/harvard/how-addiction-hijacks-the-brain.htm

Printed in Great Britain
by Amazon

61149778R00040